Did I Sign Up For This?

Did I Sign Up For This?

MARI F. HERMAN

ISBN: 1507725264
ISBN 13: 9781507725269
Library of Congress Control Number: 2015911180
Createspace Independent Publishing Platform
North Charleston, South Carolina

INTRODUCTION

Well, hello there.

Thank you for taking a peek at this book. I have to tell you now that this is not a self-help book. This is more a manuscript of questions, along with my bewilderment on why the older generation of women didn't give us ladies a heads-up of what was going to happen to us as we aged, raised children, and ventured into pregnancy, marriage, menopause, and more. If life hands me lemons, sometimes I don't want to make lemonade, dammit! I'd like to wallow in my self-pity a while, please.

So, if you are looking for a self-help book, put this back on the shelf and move on. If you are wondering what it's like to get old and have wild, crazy-ass chin hairs and other fun symptoms of getting older, then this is the book for you.

Life is hard. Accept this and move on.

The Beginning

When I was growing up, my grandmother always said I should write a book about my life. Well, I didn't feel the need to write about all that crazy, bad shit. Frankly, all people have some bad experiences in their lives, and that is what defines us. If you are a strong person, you can suck it up and move on with your life; if not, you'll wallow in self-pity and never find joy in the simple things life can offer. I am one of those people who suck it up, forgive, and move on. I'm not saying I forgive easily and accept change easily but I do give it a good effort and with time I do become the bigger person and move on. There is opportunity, however, to share life experiences that could help others. This is what I think should be told: experiences from older generations that will help make life a little easier and not so surprising when the crazy events in life happen.

Aging happens to all of us. Even if we protest, it will not listen. We all just age differently, some better than others. It's funny to see people who you went to high school with, twenty years later, and think, "She did not age well!" Come on, people, we all do that. The older I get the more I look at young ladies and can't help but wonder, "Was I like that?" Yep, that's what all older people say. They also say "back in my day." And, OMG, I am saying that! Shoot me now! I do have a sign on my desk at work that says, "Thank you for not being perky." I think that's very appropriate at this stage of my life.

Well, I am going to be fifty in a few weeks (I'm crying as I think about it), and I often wonder why my grandmothers and my two mothers (I have a stepmom and a biological mom) didn't warn me about the womanly changes that I should watch out for. As a young lady, I didn't imagine my body changing like it has. The younger generation is super lucky that women my age are more open to talk to them about everything! I mean, back when Dr. Ruth talked about s-e-x that was "sinful," women didn't talk about such things! If they did, women whispered about it. So, if you are still with me, let's take a little trip through some of my memories. If this didn't happen to you, just bear with me.

I never thought I would be fifty like I said, I thought my life and my body would be a perfect little package. Boy was I wrong. Life is not perfect. There's crazy shit that happens, and it can be a wild ride. Maybe if the older generation would have said, "Hey, life is crazy! Hold onto your ass!" I would have paid better attention. Maybe not, but hey it would have been worth the shout out.

I remember when I was a little girl I saw my great-grandmother wearing very thick stockings. Curious, I asked my great-grandmother (Sister Hunter) about it. Her answer was, "It's nothing you need to worry about. Grandma is fine." Well, turns out she had those ugly, thick stockings for varicose veins! It's not just varicose veins that are a problem but the creepy spider veins, they sneak up on you. Thanks for telling me that those things get passed on and maybe I should take better care of my legs, like wearing supportive pantyhose when I'm working and standing on my feet all day. So, I didn't protect myself, and now you can map out a trip from Lodi to Los Angeles on my legs. I am going to blame this on McDonald's® and the long hours I put in standing on my feet cooking all the fabulous food. Why not? Everyone blames McDonald's® these days. Looking back over the years I remember watching my Grandma Mimi and her sisters take tweezers to each other's faces. It was kind of funny to watch my aunts and Mimi do this. They all wore glasses and ended up yelling at each other. Picture the scene from *My Big Fat Greek Wedding*. I never paid much attention to what they were doing. I just went about playing with my brothers. Do you think any of those old ladies said anything like, "Hey pay attention kid because you're gonna get these stray, freaky hairs on your face when you are older." Nope, not a word. Thanks, ladies! So as I'm gazing in the mirror, getting ready for work in the morning, I often think, "Holy shit, what happened?!" Is this normal wear and tear on the body? What is really going on here? Some people age better than others, for sure, but do they like their aging process? I don't! Did my grandmas and mothers take it better than me? I don't know, they never talked about aging. Would I have listened to my elders if they actually told me a few things about life's little ups and downs, or would I have just heard "blah, blah, blah" and thought to myself, "They're full of shit." I guess I'll never know. Maybe we should really think about all the stuff that women have to go through like how to properly shave your legs, boys and dating, marriage, pregnancy, children, "empty-nest syndrome," menopause, and aging gracefully.

READY SET GO

Alrighty then, shaving your legs. I am half-German, half-Russian. So, I am quite hairy. Not like mountain woman weed-whacker hairy, just your normal German hairy. So in the sixth grade, I wanted to shave my nasty, hairy legs. My stepmother, Rose, said "of course." She didn't give me any instructions, just, "Soap up your legs and be careful." Okay, I can do that. Any guesses on how that worked?! Not so well. Cut the hell out of my legs, all the way up the shin, the part with the least amount of skin on the bone. I still have the scars to prove it. So, a little instruction would have been totally nice! I still to this day on occasion cut my legs shaving and silently swear. Just to be clear, I had my stepdaughter use Nair®. SO much easier, and she had very little hair—lucky her! None of my friends shaved their legs because they had very little hair; they were no help.

READY FOR DATING?

Now that I have shaved my legs, I think I am ready for boys and maybe a little dating. To tell the truth, I really wasn't interested in boys until I was a freshman in high school. I was too busy being a tomboy and playing sports. All my friends had boyfriends in Middle School so I would do it too but wasn't very impressed with the whole boyfriend thing at that age. I had two brothers growing up, and all their friends came over. We lived in the country, so all my girlfriends were tomboys too. We played football, baseball, rode bikes, played in the creek, chased bulls, and threw cow patties at each other. And yes, we were told to go play outside and don't come home until it was dark. It was such a great time. Kids nowadays can't go outside for long periods of time and be safe like I did. I think it's a real shame. I know people say it all the time, "When I was a kid I walked a mile in the snow." Yeah, yeah…but for us it was true! We walked to catch the bus, and if we missed it, we walked about a mile down the road to catch the next bus. Yep, in the rain. My stepmom thought it built character to walk in the rain. Maybe so, I don't know. Okay, I am off subject. Back to boys! Boys and girls in high school are weird. They really shouldn't date. We are all just finding out about our bodies, hormones, and personalities. I probably could have used a little more insight in this of course. Dating is a process. I don't know how it is now, but back when I was younger, it was going to the movies, bowling, skating, and you always went as a group. Just holding hands was good and hanging out. That was better—less pressure, more people to talk to. My first "car date" was at sixteen, and well, there was the awkward silence. What do you say?! Someone could have given me some clues on what to say. I mean we were in high school, not like we were worldly. The expectations of dating should be that the boy or man should always open doors for us ladies. I don't care what generation we are in—that should never change. If the two discuss how the date should go and spilt the cost, opening the door should never be negotiated. The date is basically getting to know what each person is about, likes and dislikes. Dating should be a fun experience and not rushed. What I would tell young girls today is don't dumb yourself down for a boy! It's good to be smart, and if you are smarter than him, oh well! Anyways, moving on to the good-night kiss and the anticipation of what it is going to be like. Is it a peck on the cheek or a quick kiss on the lips? Do you use tongue?? What do you do? Grandma, mom, ANYONE?! Well, for me, the quick peck was good enough. My first kiss was in eighth grade, at a dance and the song playing was *Tonight's the Night* by Rod Stewart. The guy stuck his tongue in my mouth. I wanted to throw up! No one told me about that. Thanks, ladies! Truth be told, I am still not a fan of this. Nowadays, I see that girls are more aggressive as far as kissing, making the move on boys more than boys with girls. I know, I sound so old, but when I was younger, the girls were more shy, and the boys did all the aggressive behavior. Has our openness with the young ladies made them more aggressive and less caring about their own bodies and mind?

At this time in a young person's life, body image is super important. All my friends were wearing bras in the sixth grade. Not me! I got training bras just so I could have a bra under my shirt. I didn't like them, but you know you have to fit in. At Science Camp we had to take a shower with other girls and of course they all had boobs so guess who got made fun of? You guessed it. It's just part of being a kid which can suck. For my first real bra shopping I had to drag my poor dad with me to get them. He was such a trooper. In high school, I was called the "President of the Itty Bitty Titty Committee." That's not so nice. Thank you to the boys in my school! They were so mature. But I was very thin, maybe eighty to ninety pounds, and if you turned me sideways and I stuck out my tongue, I looked like a zipper. It's kinda funny now. Anyways, the "high school dating years" are important to a young girl, and maybe a little more direction and words of wisdom would have helped. Boys, dating, and the high school years can really test you, and you get to see who your real friends are. I would not do the high school years over again, it's tough and I think it gets tougher with every generation as the world changes and becomes more stressful.

WHAT IS LOVE?

Has anyone ever really been told what love is? I know for a fact that no one explained love to me and what it truly is. I know I love my family, friends, and pets—but what is love? There's a big difference between love and lust, and I believe that is what's happening to young adults today. Many think that if they have s-e-x (whispering) with someone, that is love and that's how you show it. But, no, that is not all of it. That is one way, and between two people it can be incredible. Lust is just looking at someone and thinking they are hot and you want to hop in the sack with them. After the lust is gone, there is nothing left, nothing in common, no connection other than sex. In many dictionaries, love means "strong affection." But what the hell is that? Is it the butterflies in your belly when you go out on the first date? Is it looking at that person and getting lost in their eyes? Well, I don't have the answer, and again, I guess neither did the ladies in my family. . Love is tolerance of each other; love is understanding, acceptance, and growing together. All I can say is learn to love yourself because you can't love someone else if you can't love yourself.

Saying I do

After all the dating, if you are lucky enough to find the right person, the next step is usually marriage. Make sure you want to spend the rest of your life with this person not just for right now but forever. Young kids today throw the word "love" around and think they know what it means.. They say you marry your best friend, but do you really? Do you tell that person everything you tell your girlfriend? I'm not so sure. There were no words of advice or wisdom from my grandmothers or my mothers on this subject. However, it is totally my fault that I didn't catch a clue that marriage is hard-ass work when I look back at my family. My grandma was married three times, my mom three times, my dad two, my stepmom three. Right there I should have thought, "Don't do it!" But I am my own person, and I thought I wasn't going to be like them. As it turned out, I am on marriage number two. So many little things go into the pre marriage planning, this can cause increase stress. It can make the happiest of couples not so happy. The cost of my first marriage was relatively inexpensive compared to nowadays. My dress was made for $100, and it was so pretty. The flowers, hall, food, decorations, the church, the honeymoon—that all adds up to big dollars but not mine, I am pretty frugal. My first wedding was about $5,000 total. These days that doesn't go very far. With all the planning and costs, the happy couple will end up fighting way too much. After all that stress of planning and some other crap that went wrong, I ended up eloping the second time. We went to Mervyn's and got our rings, then headed to Reno. Total cost was $400. I truly believe that if people want to get married, they should go somewhere like Reno and *then* have a big reception. Save your money for a down payment on a house or a fabulous honeymoon. But, then again, what do I know?

We got married with no money, just dreams. Now, this is okay, but it can add so much stress starting out. This is what I try to tell young people today. Learn from me, make sure it is really right and you don't have to struggle in the beginning. Starting a marriage with little or no income can be super stressful, but having a good support system can help. Lucky for me, I have a good mother-in-law who did just that. In today's society, everything is disposable including relationships. There are those who think it's easier to scrap it and start over. Some relationships are not supposed to work but if its minor stuff, and you took your vows seriously, you try your damnedest to make it work. It's not all gravy, but it just might be worth it in the end. Some days you want to pluck you spouse's eyes out, and other times you look at them and think you are the luckiest person in the world.

After the wedding and honeymoon, you come home and have to settle into married life, life of just the two of you getting to know each other. By getting to know each other, and I mean *really* knowing them, like their annoying, bad habits that when you were dating, you let go of and thought they were so cute. Marriage means to be one, and to be one means you have to share. Now, no one, and I mean no one, told me I had to share! I flunked that in kindergarten. I am not a good sharer. I hate it. I'm the oldest child and we do not share well at all! I don't want to share my bowl of popcorn, ice cream, or toothbrush. And no, I don't want to share my side of the bed either.

When you first get married, you will turn a blind eye to a lot of things that your beloved spouse does, and at some point in the marriage these things will make you absolutely bonkers. Everything is fun and new. But as the months turn to years, things change and begin to bother you. This happens because you are not only lovers and friends, now you are partners and roommates. You're comfortable with each other but also need some time to yourself, to be with the person you lost when two became one. There will be times when you don't want to be attached at the hip and actually want to be with your friends or just in your own space. That's totally fine and very natural. I know

I have these feelings from time to time. I'm not going to lie. One time my husband asked, "What's your problem?" My reply was, "My problem?! My problem is you are still breathing!" Now, that's a little harsh, but at the time it sounded good. Also, I have to admit it was the beginning of menopause, but that's another subject to come later. Some things were overlooked in the beginning, like leaving the toilet seat up, putting dishes in the sink and not in the dishwasher, which is right next to the sink for God's sake, or thinking their stinky-ass fart is funny. *No*, I don't think that farting and then fanning out the blankets so I can smell it is funny! The list can go on and on. I'm sure there are plenty of things that bug the shit out of him about me, but I don't care about that at this moment, this is about me. Marriage is a partnership, but it may not always be equal. Men think it's equal. There will always be someone in the relationship that does more than the other. Some men think if they pick their underwear up off the floor, their work is done for the day, or if they actually pee in the toilet instead of around it, they helped because you don't have to clean the pee off the floor. Me, I'm just happy if the dishes actually get *in* the dishwasher. Don't be like me and try to be "Super wife" in the beginning and wait on your man, clean the house, and go to work. I did it all and spoiled the crap out of him. So, when I actually needed help because I was so tired of doing it all, he was shocked and didn't know what to do. This was the point in the marriage that I snapped. He was surprised that I actually needed help with the house or anything else. My husband didn't get it at first when I started complaining and snapping at him that I could not do it all. Now he knows when I get that look in my eye, he better help. Not all spouses are this way. Some of you are very lucky and have the most fabulous man that is actually your equal and will help with all the laundry, washing dishes, cooking, and all the other little chores that a woman does. I have family and friends who are lucky enough to find that person who will go shopping with them, cook, and help clean. Those men are few and far between.

Like I said before, some of us don't get it right the first time. That's me. I have been married now for twenty years on marriage number two. Marriage is like the wedding ring, a full circle. That's what the relationship becomes. In the beginning you overlook little things, in the middle things make you nuts, and now you are back to a more tolerance of each other. You actually share, you are better friends, and it's just you two again. The children have grown and have possibly left and started their lives and you have time for each other. The feeling of butterflies in your belly goes away through the years and instead you develop a friendship, a comfortable relationship for both of you. Yep, I actually share now. Not everything, but I share. I tell all the young ladies and boys that I know, including my own kids, that marriage is hard-ass work. Even if you find that person you think is wonderful and perfect, it is still hard work and no one is perfect, including me. (Wow that was hard to get out.) So much responsibility goes into marriage. You're both learning about each other, and there are outer stressors that put weight on your shoulders that can cause a big kink in the marriage. There are jobs, bills, upkeep on the cars and house, and the children. Children are a huge stressor, especially teenagers. What I tell young people is be real certain that you want to get married. Make sure you have a job to help pay all the bills. Money problems can strain even the strongest of marriages. Continue to have time for you. Encourage each other to be the best you both can be and then build from there. Push each other every day to be better people. When you fight, try not to say hurtful things to each other. You can forgive, but those words stay with you for a long time, and eventually the marriage will breakdown. Apologize when you are wrong. Just suck it up and do it. Don't take each other for granted. This doesn't always happen on purpose—it just happens. Life can get really busy, especially if you have children. Make sure you find time to spend with just the two of you. Couples can grow in different directions, and that's normal. However, you have to find a way to be with each other and remember the couple who fell in love and wanted to spend the rest of your lives together. Find a way to have the same interests or at least compromise and share the interest of your partner. It's okay to have different interests and friends, but the key is to find quality time with each other. Marriage is love, tolerance, sharing, compromise, understanding, and some sex thrown in for good measure. Marriage is like a roller coaster, ups, downs, excitement and then the calm. As I heard some-where, marriage isn't happily ever after; it's a contract to grow together. It is hard work, but through that work you will have love. If my grandmothers and mothers would have told me a few of these things, maybe marriage number one wouldn't have happened or turned out differently. Or I could have heard "blah, blah, blah," and did what I wanted anyway. No one knows.

Sex and Marriage

Should we talk a little about sex in marriage? So, sex is part of the whole relationship. But when the communication breaks down due to stressors in your life, sex can take a back seat. It's the last thing on your mind. This can cause you both to get mad and then grow further apart. Once you grow apart, it's harder to get back in the groove of things, and the marriage will begin to fail. The bond for men in the relationship is sex. Now, it may not be that for all men, but for most it's sex. For men, they think when you have sex everything is so much better when in fact it may not be. Women want intimacy as well as the problems to be fixed. To women, sex does not fix the problems; it helps make things go away for about a five minutes (she said jokingly), then it's back to worry and stress. Men think sex heals or fixes everything while women think that talking things through is the way. Men are not talkers; they just need to know the basics. Again, this is not all men, just the ones I have encountered. We know that as women we make most of the decisions—furniture, paint colors, household stuff, kid issues and day to day stuff. We just let the men think they are making most of the decisions or helping. So, men think if you aren't having sex with them, you either don't love them or you're cheating. Now, we know this isn't true, but men are insecure. In the beginning there will be lots of sex; however that will change with time. As the years go by some things are just as good, like holding hands, watching a movie on the couch, sharing and enjoying each other's company. With that being said, there will be days when you feel totally ugly, fat, and/or gassy, and he will say, "Hey, baby, go put something sexy on." In my mind, I'm thinking, "Great, nothing fits me that is remotely sexy. I'm too gassy and bloated to even think about sex right now." I just want to take a tummy pill and lie down alone! But you have to remember your man doesn't care about all those things; he is only thinking "Boobs!" Don't get me wrong, I like sex just as much as anyone else, but sometimes after a hard day at work, dealing with kids and everything else, it's difficult to get in that mindset. There may be days where you just want to watch a movie, and then he does the whole hungry eyes thing at you. What do you do? Well, I play "beat the popcorn." I tell my man, "Look, I really wanted to settle in and watch a movie, so you got till the microwave popcorn is done." Yep, that did happen. And when kids come along, he has until SpongeBob is done. I have many fond memories of SpongeBob.

Just SEX

My biological mother did tell me a little about sex. She asked me if I knew what a penis was. I told her yep, and she said "Great, stay away from it." Words of wisdom right there.

I am no Dr. Ruth, but I have observed some things about sex in my years. Sex is something that is learned. No one shares the do's and don'ts with you. You learn by default. Some women are more in tune to their body and know what they want and how to get it. My generation and previous generations did not talk about sex—as I have mentioned earlier. The problem with the current culture is they use sex as a way to get the person they want, or they're too casual about the whole act. It has been evolving since the '80s, when people would go to clubs and have one night stands. But now it is extreme; children are having sex. Children as young as twelve are having sex and babies. Do they even know what they are doing? Do they really understand what they were doing, or are they trying to be cool? Having casual sex or having many partners doesn't make you an expert about it. It doesn't mean you know your body or are a great lover. It just makes you sexually active with way too many partners and that isn't a good thing, but this is just my opinion. It's about respecting your body and making sure the person you are intimate with is going to be there for you for more than three minutes, three hours, or three years. It's about a lifetime together. This is something that may have been good to know as an adolescent. So, that is a little off subject however I am struggling with the whole casual sex with this generation that is among us. I just want to scream at them and say "What the hell are you thinking?"

Some women can talk dirty or are loud during sex. I am not one of them. I just can't do it. It sounds ridiculous to me when I say it out loud. I can think it sometimes, but talk dirty without giggling—not so much. They say a man wants a nice woman to take care of the house, children, and other day-to-day living and then be a hooker in the bedroom. Well, do *we* actually want to do that? I'm not too sure about that concept. Is anyone else? I don't really know about this because, again, this is not a topic that ladies want to discuss. Ladies, we know that porn is just porn and men like to watch porn, but why do they want to try what they see on TV? "Put some spice in the relationship," he says. I'm thinking you want spice, baby, let me get the oregano out of the cabinet and sprinkle it on you—there's your spice! There are different stages of sex, some people say. They say that you can be sexually active well into your eighties. I'm not sure I want to. I am a nurse, and I've seen the aging population naked. It's not pretty. Hugh Hefner had kids in his seventies! I have to wonder if he uses Viagra, and what the hell is his wife thinking?!

With sex comes being comfortable with your body and knowing how to achieve the goal—an orgasm. Yep, I said the word orgasm! This is a learned process. No one I knew even mentioned the word orgasm—yikes! Well, Dr. Ruth did and, oh boy, did people get upset. As you get older (by that, I mean late thirties and more mature), I think you know your body more and you want more pleasure out of the act of sex. Some young girls may already be at this point, but my generation, I don't think we were. I think we were more reserved and willing to let the man take over. Having sex at a young age, like in your teens, I don't think you are physically or mentally mature enough. I don't think that girls today even really know what sex is supposed to be. What is it suppose to be you might ask. Well, it's between two adults who are in a committed relationship and all that comes with it. Not just a casual hookup. That just leaves one person feeling sad and alone. There is too much stuff on TV, on the Internet, and in books that makes things more glamorous than in real life. The point I am trying to make is that a person, whether a boy or girl, should be both physically and mentally mature before they venture into the world of sex. Now, God plays a mean trick on us. Women mature more quickly than men. So, we become mentally mature, but are we physically mature? That is tough question to measure. They say men will peak sexually in their twenties and women in their thirties and forties. There is something wrong with this picture. I don't think boys and men mature mentally until they are well into their forties and fifties. Like Judge Judy says, "After that, it's all downhill." It's at this age that you might want sex more than you did when you were younger, and you begin actually telling your man you want sex. So, when you finally want sex (without him making the first move) and tell him what you want it, he will be in shock. Of course, this may throw your man overboard because this is new to him. He is used to making the moves and you being passive and just going with the flow. As you mature, you bond more with your husband, and you feel more comfortable telling him what you want and how you're feeling. You're more comfortable in your skin as the saying goes. It does take a little adjusting on his part, but in the end, I think he will like the new you. As you mature and blossom, you feel more comfortable and begin to enjoy some of the changes your body is going through. I am still struggling with the fact that my body is changing. I wonder if my husband is going to still want me as I age. Like I said earlier, I'm a nurse. I see older people and I'm not sure I want to go there naked! By then, being romantic might have to be with candlelight romantic setting in the *other* room! So, you have self-confidence when you are young with your body, but when you are older you have self-confidence with sex but not necessarily your body. No one said any of these things to me. These are things I have learned and observed over the years. If people out there are lucky enough for the older generation to give them little talks about sex, body changes, and all that other really juicy stuff, they are lucky. Do you talk to your friends about your body changes and sexual acts? Have you ever asked them, "Hey, are you feeling more sexual as you get older?" "Is the Big O more intense? 'Cause mine is, and it's awesome!" Really, how much do you say to your friends? Do they feel the same about sex and orgasms? I think *Cosmo* magazine is a big help in times of need. Like, during sex, is it normal for a woman's mind to wonder?

Did I Sign Up For This?

Has this happened to anyone else? And I don't mean you start thinking about another man, just other things, like how much laundry you have to do, or what's for dinner, those kinds of things. It's not a bad thing, or is it? Or is it just that we have so much on our plates to juggle that our minds wander? I wonder what men think about. Of course when you ask they say, "I'm thinking of you, baby." They are probably thinking of you for a minute, and then it's on to Pam Anderson.

Anyway, sex is what you make of it. It is good for a healthy marriage. Make it all that it can be to satisfy you and your man, whatever it takes to keep you both on the same page. Communicate with your spouse and keep the lines of communication open. Remember, sex is healthy, helps burn calories, and relieves stress!

CHILDREN ANYONE?

While we're on the subject of sex, I guess I should mention some stuff about pregnancy and children. As a couple, you decide you are ready for kids—oh boy! Sometimes it takes longer, and the couple "has to practice" more. I remember when my husband and I decided the time was right. During the act of making a baby the phone rang. We let the answering machine pick up; of course it was my in-laws. Afterward, my husband called back, and I hear him say, "We were making you another grandchild." Then my husband yells, "Mom says to keep your legs and butt up for half an hour." Geez!!!

Looking back, my grandmothers and mothers never really mentioned anything about being pregnant or raising kids. Their famous line was, "You just wait." Wait?! What the hell for? Give me some insight, please!

Anyways, you are now pregnant and hopefully going through the best experience in your life, and it's supposed to be the most beautiful thing in the world. Most pregnant women have "the glow." I found the glow about five months into it. The first few months, your body is changing so much. I didn't really focus on it because I was pretty nauseated. I worked in a hospital with some pretty funky smells especially lunch trays! But everyone is different with her symptoms. Everyone will tell you stories about being pregnant and about the delivery. Mostly it's the horrible delivery stories and the pain. Why do they wait until you are already knocked up?! I could have used this knowledge prior to having a little alien suck the life right out of me. All kidding aside, I was the healthiest I had ever been when I was pregnant. I have lupus, and they weren't sure I could get pregnant. It did take about a year (although my husband says a month), but it was a year. When pregnant, we ladies need to eat healthy so our little bundle of joy can grow. For me, I started to "show" at nine weeks, and I was very ill. I had no idea I was pregnant because my doctors told me it couldn't happen. By three months I was wearing very large clothes and could not see my feet or my "who who." Since everyone is different while pregnant, you should never compare what you are going through to someone else and think that something is wrong with you. Lucky for me, there were twelve of us pregnant at the same time and all with boys but one. It was great because being in the health care profession we could ask those questions that we are generally afraid to ask. Like, does it feel like someone is pulling on your labia? (Yep, I said it.) Are my boobs supposed to look like this? Does it feel like a foot is gonna come out of your vagina? Is it normal to want sex more now than when I wasn't pregnant? And yes, for some women, they want sex more. The reason there is more blood flow down in that area and it makes it more sensitive, that's the nurse version. All the questions you have are valid, yet you can't ask people you don't know. The good thing about being pregnant is the big boobs (unless you already have big boobs), but then your belly is also big. Let's talk about your boobs and pregnancy for a minute. What no one mentions is that your pre pregnancy perky boobs will no longer be that way after you have your bundle of joy. Those once fabulous, firm boobs will be a pile of mush. So not only did your bundle of joy suck the life out of you for nine months, it takes your boobs. Now, mine were not big by all means, but they were perky, and I liked them. Of course the bigger the belly the more of a challenge when you actually want sex. Finding the right angle and position, you have to be creative. I wanted sex, and my husband was like, "Are you kidding me?!" I didn't care how big I was. I wanted it, and he better damn well make it happen!

So, when pregnant, it's normal to have morning sickness. That means you have more hormones. Hormones are a scary thing. So many mood swings. One minute you are happy, then sad or crying or just plain bitchy. Family and friends beware. Some nursing tips that I found helpful, drink more water than coffee and soda as these have caffeine and can cause dehydration. I learned that and felt so much healthier and better the more water I drank. Walk a lot for good cardio. The more fit you are the better labor is supposed to be. If your belly is big like mine was, I found that rubbing lotion (any lotion) on it every night helped with stretch marks. Don't scratch! Rub. This being said, some people are prone to stretch marks, and others are not. Some positive points on having a big belly is you can rest your midnight snack on it, and people let you have their seat in busy cafes and public transportation. However, since you can't see your toes or bend over to even polish your toes, you have a good excuse to get pedicures more often. The sucky thing is you can't shave your legs, and if you happen to shave or groom in other areas that proves to be a challenge, unless of course your man will do that for you. Mine, not so much. Let's take a quick minute to talk about grooming your "lady parts." Some ladies have more than their share of excess hair, others do not. Some like to wax it totally off or make designs. I think just keeping it neatly groomed and not having it come out from your panties is a good idea. I have to wonder what the past generations did about grooming or if it was a taboo. But again, grooming is totally up to you, and again, my elders never told about this so it was something I actually had to learn about and did on my own because I don't like messy or hanging out everywhere! So, heads up, you may go into labor with the "native look." Embarrassing!

The birthing classes are a must. They help with focusing through the contractions. You don't need to go with every pregnancy but at least the first so you learn the technique. For some it is beneficial, some not. I thought it was a huge help. Unfortunately, for me, my focal point happened to be my husband's face. At this stage of the game I really didn't want to look at him. I was irritated at him, but if I didn't look at him, I couldn't breathe through the contractions. He would get tired of me looking at him and try to move away, which turned out bad for him. He said, "I can't stay in that position and look at you the whole time." Really?! I told him, "It's not about you, and you will do it!" Rule to remember: Don't piss off the pregnant lady.

Pregnancy is a special time, and it should be a happy one. Everyone's pregnancy is different so enjoy yours and remember you have a beautiful human growing in your belly.

Did I Sign Up For This?

Let's talk about the birth process. First, people say when you get that "nesting" feeling, you're close to delivery, and they are so right. I thought it meant that you got into a cleaning phase. Well, it can be anything. For me, I focused on the damn stroller. It was three weeks before my due date, and I was trying to put the stroller together. I could not get the axle on, and I had a complete meltdown. I called the hubby, and he told me to wait until he got home from work. Of course I am full on in tears and breaking down. I called my sister-in-law who was very pregnant with her fourth child. She came right over. She was a pro at getting these things together and promptly told me I would have that baby soon because I was so focused on the stroller. I went to the doctor the next day, and she said I was dilated to two and it would be any-time from a few days to a week. Well, that night I went into labor. If you are pregnant for the first time and go into labor, here are a few tips. If you feel like you have menstrual cramps all day - that is labor. No one told me this includ-ing my doctor. I had menstrual-like cramping the whole day when I got back from the doctor. She told me to continue walking. I tried to take our old dog for a walk and had to keep stopping. I only made it to the corner and had to come back. The dog kept looking at me like "Hey, what the hell?" That should have been a clue, but I didn't catch on. When my husband got home from work, I told him I felt like I was going to start my period. He laughed and said, "Have you looked in the mirror? You are very pregnant and huge." Well, of course I know I'm very pregnant. I can't see my feet, asshole! Later on, I had just settled into bed, found a comfortable position and *wham*, I had to pee again! I was so mad. When I got up, I thought I had peed my pants. It was all over the floor, which made me even more upset. Then it dawned on me—my water just broke. Then panic set in. Holy shit, I am not due for three weeks, and my water broke. I'm not packed. I'm not ready! I went into the bathroom to clean myself up and the mess on the floor. Of course, it didn't stop. I called the hospital and was told I had lots of time, and since it was my first baby, I should come in when I felt the contractions more often. Well, I didn't feel contractions; I only felt menstrual cramps that weren't too bad. (I have a high tolerance for pain.) This was at 11:00 p.m. I woke the hubby, got dressed, and called my mother-in-law to come stay with my stepdaughter. We left and got to the hospital around midnight. The house supervisor, who I knew very well, asked how far apart the contractions were. I told her I didn't know because they were too mild to tell. So she calculated. They were one minute apart. I never saw anyone move so fast. She thought I was going to have the baby in the elevator! When I got to the OB unit, they took me right in and had me put on the hospital gown. Then they did the cruelest thing they can do to any hormonal woman in labor—they had me step on the scale. I started to cry when I saw the weight, ugh! I was 155 pounds. When I got pregnant, I was 105 pounds. So, they put me in the bed, started the IV, and hooked the baby up to monitors. This was the fun part. The contractions start kicking in, and the husband is watching the monitor saying, "Here comes one." God love him, he was so excited and thought he was helping. Of course I say, "No shit, I can feel it!" They actually weren't that bad. I tell the hubby, "If I would have known that this was it, I would have done this a long time ago." Then Mother Nature steps in, and you suddenly have to pee and poop, her way of making room for the baby to come out without you pooping all over the table or the hospital staff which is exactly what I was thinking. The contractions are coming; the nurse says she will give me a mild pain reliever because I appear uncomfortable. She gives me Toradol. After, she asks me how I feel. I tell her, "Like I just smoked a big, fat one." Okay, probably not the brightest thing to say since I am a nurse, I work here, and I don't do drugs. I dabbled when I was younger, but I am a lightweight with even Motrin. Well, about a half hour into this, I tell the nurse I have to push. She checks, and sure enough, I am kinda ready but there is part of my cervix in the way and she has to hold it open at the top and tells me I can't push. Whatever, I am pushing to get that thing out of me! My body has totally taken over, and the contractions are doing all the work. I have lost control, and all I can think about is "Please, God, don't let me poop on the table, I work with these people." Well, as it turned out, the kid got stuck after the third push, and it was all downhill from there. Lucky for me, I don't remember anything after that but a few details. I remember being on the gurney, and the nurse putting in the spinal, them strapping me down to the OR table, and me waking up saying, "He's not breathing." Now mind you, I didn't know if I was having a boy or a girl, and I didn't see the baby because I was too out of it, but I knew it was a boy. Months prior, I had a dream that I was on an operating room table and I had a boy. My dream came true; it was exactly like my dream. People told me that if you dream about a boy or girl, that's what you will have, and sure enough it's true. The nurses were fabulous, and the nursery nurse taught me how to breast-feed effectively. Breast-feeding is not for everyone, however the baby's poop does not stink with breast feeding, and that's a plus! I chose to breastfeed because of how sick my son was and it helped him. I did breast feed for twelve weeks and then switched to the bottle because I had to go back to work. Once I gave him the bottle he didn't want the boob! Bottle comes out faster so he would refuse the boob. I had enough milk for five babies and he wouldn't take it! It was a huge milky mess every time I tried to give him my boob. Well, then I pumped, showed him! There are pros and cons with breast feeding and it's up to you to do what is best for you and your baby. Basically, the point of this super long rant is everyone's birthing experience is very different.

After you give birth, a tip I think is very important is to sleep as much as the baby for the first few weeks. You need to let the housework and laundry go, or have someone help. If you try to clean and do all the wife stuff when the baby is napping, you will become sleep deprived and that's when you become grumpy and postpartum depression will set in. I tried to be Superwoman when my son came home. I still did all the chores around the house and was running on fumes. I became an emotional wreck, crying all the time. The doctor laughed and told me to take naps and go on walks outside with the baby to get some vitamin D in me. Well, that worked, and I try to tell all new moms to do this. Good tip! Exercise increases endorphins which makes you happy and happy people don't kill people. The doctor also told me to avoid sex for four to six weeks. No worries there, I am rethinking this whole sex thing!

Also, another tip to remember during pregnancy that I totally forgot is to do your Kegel exercises. I have seen this with many women, and yet again this was not mentioned to me. Some woman will have stretched ligaments from child rearing, which later on will cause the ligaments to become weak, which in turn will cause the bladder to prolapsed or cause leaking. (This is probably a little too much nursing information, but my mom's never told me about this). Now, it doesn't happen all the time, however I have been noticing that when I sneeze, I feel like I might pee my pants. So, try to do your Kegel exercises as much as possible. Keep those muscles healthy. This will keep the vagina (I said it again!) nice and tight so when it gets stretched out it, will go back again. I'm doing them now—ha-ha! All kidding aside, as you get older have this talk with your physician if you feel like you are having stress incontinence or leaking. Make sure you do the Kegels after pregnancy too. Your husband will appreciate this. I'm mentioning this because my stepdaughter is pregnant, and I forgot to tell her this. But lucky for me she is a bright girl and remembered on her own.

Don't let other people's stories of pregnancy, birth process, and taking care of the baby scare you. Yours will be what it is for you, your hubby, and the whole family. Enjoy having a new life growing inside of you and after the delivery.

Bringing the Bundle
of Joy Home

I have a stepdaughter—and I didn't have to deliver her. So much easier than delivery, and she was potty trained—yahoo! She was so easy thought I should try this pregnancy, birth, and potty-training thing—what was I thinking?! I had a traumatic delivery, which lucky for me I don't remember, but my poor husband has now had two traumatic deliveries. I think I will blame all the birthing problems on him because I can. So, now it's time to bring the baby home. This is a time of bonding. It can be a great time. The first day home can be interesting. You don't have the nurses there to help with the little tot, but I had my mother-in-law, which was good. However, she did get a huge surprise from the little bundle of joy. I had just finished breast-feeding, and the kid ate for a good half hour. I forgot to burp him during and after, and as I handed him to my poor mother-in-law, he projectile vomited all over her and the couch! I was totally mortified. She was a trooper.

Watching your little baby every day and seeing all the things they learn is super fun. They are so fun and loving as little babies and toddlers. Their brains are like little sponges taking in all their surroundings and wanting to learn. It is a learning process for us parents as well. Like, do you try to use the binky or not? Well, my son was a five-binky baby. At night, he had one in each hand, one in his mouth, and two at the end of the crib so if he lost one I could quickly replace it. I am a sleep lover so I do need my sleep, and when you have to work the next morning, it's hard to be up all night with a fussy baby. Everyone told me to break him of that habit because he would have to have braces. I thought, do I pay for braces later and stay happy, or take the binky away and be miserable? Well, I chose happy baby, happy mommy. When I finally decided to take the binky away when he was about one, he spoke for the first time. It was his own language, but he talked. He did speak little words but not good, I later learned that he could not hear from fluid in his ears and had to have tubes. The first few nights without the binky were very hard, I won't lie. One night, my husband, my stepdaughter, and I were watching TV, and my son was in his crib without his binky. When he woke up, we could hear him say, "Where's my binky?" But he said it very loudly and in a voice like Regan from *The Exorcist*. Scared the crap out of all of us, and my husband said, "Go check on him and make sure his head isn't spinning." He was scared to go in there—big pansy! It took a good week for him go to sleep without a binky fight. After a year had passed, I was moving furniture and moving his crib. My son came in the room, and at the same time we both spied a binky under the crib. I tell you what; we both dove at the same time to get that binky. Luckily, the little nipple part was broke off so he couldn't put it in his mouth. I still have that binky.

The first cold can be scary, as well as the first ear infection and all the other diseases that come along. I was good at ear infections because my step-daughter had a lot of them. My son was sick a lot. He was born severely sick, and it lasted for the first five years, his tonsils were so big and were always getting infected-yuk! He had lots of fevers while he was teething. Because of the fevers it burned the enamel on his teeth. So the permanent teeth that came in had brown spots. Here are a few things about kids being sick. It's a struggle. My stepdaughter used to get ear infections, and I remember being up long nights with her until she had tubes put in. My son had lots of very high fevers (up to 105) with him being very lethargic so I have learned a few tips. When a child is teething, elevate the crib a little. You can roll up a towel, blanket, or something like that under the mattress at the head of the bed, this is a tip I learned the hard way. Nurse information again-the baby's Eustachian tubes (tubes in the ears) are horizontal, and the fluids don't drain. These tubes will be vertical around age four or five. So, with the head elevated, the fluid will drain instead of collecting, which causes infection. If you happen to get a sick baby, humidifiers, or Vicks plug-ins really help, and now they have the baby Vicks rub in patches you can stick on their chest. It's the best thing ever for stuffy noses. Also, try not to have your baby go on antibiotics too much because they will build up a resistance, and if you can give a probiotic with the antibiotics, it will help to prevent diarrhea. Antibiotics will take all the good bacteria out of their little bellies with the bad bacteria. For fevers, use Tylenol and alternate with Motrin. But remember, some fevers are okay because it means the body is trying to fight the infection. Of course a fever of 104–105 like my son warrants a call to the doctor or trip to the ER. For a fussy, gassy baby, a trick I learned from my mother-in-law is to put the baby on its back and bring an arm and the opposite leg and have them meet at the belly. Do this to the other arm and leg, then take your hands and place them under the baby's back, and use your thumbs to rub gentle circles on baby's belly. The baby will let out the gas. Do this a few times. Also, the bottles made to decrease the gas work great.

Time flies, and your child is now a toddler, learning the word "no." Awesome, right?! Do the "time outs" really work? I don't think so. People nowadays believe it's all about the time outs and no spanking. I truly think that spanking isn't bad and having a little fear of your parents is okay. I have no advice or little tricks about toddlers. They are still learning, and they will challenge you because they can, same as teenagers. If they happen to be afraid of the dark, you might do what I did. I used to tell my son that monsters are afraid of mommies and gave him a flashlight to keep by him. That seemed to do the trick.

Then the school years begin. That is a huge challenge as a parent. Peer pressure starts. As a parent, how much pressure do you put on them to get good grades, be themselves, and try to get along with all the other little monsters in their school? My son had a good heart and didn't fight back with the other kids who picked on him. So, for three years of him coming home with scratches, bruises, and stories of how the other kids hit him, I sat my son down and told him, "If someone hits you first, you hit them back. You will not get in trouble from mommy." Well, a few weeks went by, and I get a call from the school. They tell me my son is in the office for hitting another child. I go to the school, and the principal begins to tell me, "We don't condone children fighting, and your son hit another child." I asked what happened. My son replies, "He hit me in the spine so I hit him back in the spine." (A child of a nurse!) I told the principal, "There you go. My son will not be a punching bag for other students, and I will not punish him for defending himself." That was one thing my parents did help me with when I was younger. They always told me to stick up for myself and to not let other children pick on me or hit me. I got into a few fights because other kids did hit me and tried to pick on me, but I held my ground. That was a lesson that was good for me, and I did pass that one. No one should be bullied.

Then there's the homework and the after-school activities that will keep you pretty busy. If you have time, helping in the classroom is very rewarding, and you get to see how your child does with others, as well as how effective the teachers are. Then come the teen years—middle school and high school. I think the girl was so much easier than the boy. Girls dealing with peer pressure, body changes, and hormones can be a challenge, and children nowadays are very cruel. My stepdaughter used to come to work with me on special occasions. I worked at a unit in the hospital that had tracheotomy and ventilator patients. Some of these patients were in vegetative states while others had significant brain damage from drugs and alcohol abuse. She got to see this, and it was a good way for her to remember it as a teen. When Chris Farley died, I heard her tell her friend, "That's what happens when you do drugs." Proud momma moment right there. The sex talk was okay. I answered all her questions honestly and told her that it's her decision since it's her body, but she needs to respect herself first. I think you have to be honest with that discussion because they are going to do what they want anyway. Remind them that sex should never be casual, be responsible and it's okay to say no. I talked about sex from my point of view and then from a nurse's because STDs are very scary and on the rise.

The boy is more of a challenge with everything because of the age difference between him and his sister (nine years). He thinks that I am his sibling and not his mother and will challenge everything I say. Also, in high school the teachers tend to be a little more liberal than I like, and my child thinks that it is a democracy in the house. He said, "Don't we live in America? Don't I get a say so?" I have to remind him that it's a "Momocracy" and, no, he does not get a vote. I have no helpful tips for the teen years other than be as honest as possible with questions related to drugs, alcohol, and sex. Keep your child active in sports or after school activities to keep them out of mischief. Let the child know when they are being disrespectful and hurtful. Setting limits is good, and I still believe a curfew should be in place. And try super hard to not kill the child—just kidding. Going through this right now, I have to say I long for the days when I came home from work, and my son was happy to see me and wanted to talk to me. They are little for such a short time, so embrace it.

With that being said, I could go on and on about the experiences I've had with my two, but children really are your greatest joy and your greatest heartache. Enjoy what you can, pray during the bad and challenging times, and enjoy them when they really appreciate you again.

THE M WORD

I think I should also bring up menopause since it is a huge part of my life right now. After I had my son at age thirty-four, I went into early menopause. No one told me after you have children that your whole body goes through lots and lots of changes. One that comes to mind is after you have a baby your menstrual cycle changes. Your periods get really heavy. Before I had my son my period would only last a day or two. After giving birth I'd have at least two full weeks of heavy bleeding—gross! That should have given me a clue that my body was changing. With two years of crazy periods I had some crazy moods to go along with it. Then I started missing periods. I went to the doctor because I would take home pregnancy tests, and they would all be negative, but I didn't have periods. I was told nothing is wrong. After a year of dealing with this I went to an ob-gyn. She asked me how I was feeling. I told her that if I could run someone over, I would feel so much better. She said, "Okay, here is a prescription for Xanax, and let's do some lab work." Well, Xanax was a miracle drug while I waited to find out what the hell my body was going through. Turned out I was premenopausal, which meant I was starting menopause—at thirty-seven! Who knew that lupus and pregnancy would throw my body into early menopause? I also want to add that during this time I felt a constant pressure in my lower abdomen, and sex was very painful, which was not normal for me. The problem was a dry vagina (hate that word!). Guess what, now there are commercials about this everywhere! No commercials ten years ago!

Menopause is not fun. Your body will go through changes that you really don't understand. Basically, you stop producing estrogen, which your body doesn't function well without. One thing I have to say because someone else could benefit from this is I thought I was having bladder infections because it always hurt like one, especially after sex. Well, on my first exam for pre menopause, the doctor said that my bladder and vaginal walls were very dry from lack of estrogen, and if I waited any longer they would fall through, or prolapse. Yikes!!! I do remember my grandmother's uterus protruding out and she would push it back in but again nothing about this being a problem. At the time I didn't understand why and I was totally grossed out. So, then comes the fun vaginal creams and finding the right estrogen supplement that my body would respond to. Every woman has to find the right medication that works for her. Unfortunately with lupus, my body really doesn't like any medications so it was a huge challenge for my doctor. Finally, we got the right combo, and I feel somewhat human. The wacky hormones don't help this whole process. Going from wanting to kill someone to crying my eyes out was just super fun.

I can remember my stepmother with crazy mood swings, and she always had the air conditioner on in my parents' bedroom. That was the only house we lived in with an AC in the window. Back then most houses didn't have central air and heat. We had a wall heater and no AC. As a child I didn't understand what my stepmom was going through. As a woman in menopause I totally understand! I wish she would have given me a clue. I have to wonder though; did the doctors actually diagnose her right? When I first started with the symptoms, my primary care physician said, "It's stress." Nope! So, I have to imagine during the '60s, '70s, and '80s, the doctors really didn't do justice with women's health. We were all just "crazy."

Menopause brings weight gain. It's hard to lose because you crave chocolate and salt all the time just like when you were having your period. It's hard to say no to the cravings. Some women may be strong; I am not one of them. With the weight gain, the positive for me is my boobs got bigger—yippee! Husband didn't mind the weight gain because my boobs grew. So, for the first time in my adult life I actually have to dry *under* my boobs! The down side is that now I have to bend over when I put on my bra to make sure I get my entire boob in the darn thing, because as I mentioned before, they are no longer perky. However, I am not happy about the weight gain because it's mostly belly weight. I am currently trying to fix that issue, but I must not be ready because it is a slow process. I think about exercising, but then that Reese's Peanut Butter Cup looks better to me and calls me to eat it. I want to fit back into the cute clothes in my closet instead of buying a bigger size, but again the pastries and peanut butter cups are calling me.

Some woman will get adult acne too. Yep, that's me. At fifty, I have pimples and spend a crap-load of money on all sorts of acne creams. Why you ask? Well, your hormones are constantly changing so your beauty products have to change too. One product may work for a while, and then it won't. It totally sucks. Same goes for deodorants: They work for a minute, and then it's time to change—it's terrible and costly.

Sex during menopause can be interesting. Like I mentioned before, the vagina will have less secretions, mucous lining. (Nurse Talk) So, if intercourse hurts, call your doctor. Don't be shy about it either. Once you get that problem fixed, sex can be really good. Some women will have better orgasms (yep, I said it again.) I'm not sure why, but it happens. Ladies, remember your husband will be okay with a few extra pounds as long as you are having sex with him again. I say "again" because about this time, the pace you were in with your children and all their needs has hopefully slowed down and it's back to you and your partner.

Also with menopause comes crazy facial hair. Nurse talk again-due to the lack of estrogen, we now have more testosterone in our bodies so we start to get more facial hair. I am totally upset by this! I am part Russian and we are hairy people to begin with. I've begun to notice wild stray chin hairs. As a woman, if you see another woman with a crazy hair or two that they may have missed, please let them know. Don't let her go any longer with stray facial hairs! It goes against the woman code. Picture the scene from *My Big Fat Greek Wedding* where they have tweezers and they are each doing their faces. That is true sisterhood. I have no good advice on how to keep those things away: tweezing, waxing, laser hair removal—do what works for you and whatever makes you look amazing. I can say that if the world goes to shit and we have to survive like in the old days without electricity and the comforts of today, I am ready. I have my fire-starter kit, my Sally Hansen hair-remover cream (I will make it last awhile), and tweezers tucked away in an emergency take-away kit.

I do want to mention one thing though. Don't forget to have someone keep up on removing unwanted facial hair when you cannot. I mean like when you are in your eighties with dementia, make sure someone has your back. When my grandmother was dying, I went to see her at the convalescent home, and her face was a mess. She had chin, and upper lip hair and she had people coming to pray for her every day. If she was in her right mind, she wound have died from embarrassment. We are vain up until the time we are put in the grave. I removed the hair before any more visitors came, and I let the poor staff know I was pissed off and that if they see any more stray hairs they better take care of it because if it was them would they want to look like that? I have a plan B because my boy is not going to keep up on my grooming, and my stepdaughter may not live close by. I already have someone to make sure my legs are shaved and I have no crazy facial hair when I go to a convalescent home because I will have dementia when menopause is done kicking my ass.

Unfortunately, menopause never truly goes away. The night sweats and hot flashes will come and go, moods will be a challenge for the rest of your years, and family and friends will just have to understand. If they don't, then it's time for new family and new friends—just kidding. Hot flashes are super crazy. I hear ladies say, "I'm having my own private paradise." Really?! Are you friggin' kidding me? There is no paradise about it. There is no cabana boy bringing me an umbrella drink. It's more like your own private hell. You can feel this intense feeling inside, and then it's hot to the point where you can't get your clothes off quick enough. My doctor said they will go away with time. Well, ten years later they still come and go, and I have to be honest, it totally sucks.

Menopause would have been something I'd have loved my mothers and grandmothers to give me a heads-up about. I'm not sure I would have totally listened. I think back and remember my Mimi and her sisters using tweezers on their faces, my step mom with the hot flashes and crazy mood stuff I never knew why they did that and they never offered me information, maybe they did not realize it was menopause either. I literally thought my step mom was going crazy but now I get it. Maybe the doctors back then truly did not understand the whole woman process and just brushed it off as just being crazy.

More Fun Changes

Let's talk about age and extra skin. What is with the extra skin on our necks?! When I put my chin to my chest, it looks like I have three chins! I know I've gained a few pounds, but really? This is not funny. Then, in the mirror, as I am putting cream on my face and neck I noticed that I can pull the extra skin straight out. I find myself pulling at it when I am bored. I think I need a hobby. I see many women with necks that have extra skin. What do they call it? Turkey neck? Yuck. I now know why women get a tuck on their neck. Some women are just prone to this. My advice is to make sure your neck is stretched out when you have pictures taken. The back of your arm gets to swinging too! What the hell? As I shake the salt on my food, my arm shakes. When I wave, my arm waves back. Totally not right. I can't even talk about the way my butt jiggles now. There are things to fix these issues and someday I may take action. Right now I am too busy with my pity party.

Aging and menopause bring more changes with your skin. Some women may get these weird skin tags, flat clear moles, or flat dark moles that are hard that the doctors like to call barnacles (gross but my grandmother had them and I think I found one!). I used to love my chest and would wear V-neck shirts but not so much as I age.

While we are talking about aging and all the fun body changes lets also bring up the grey hair issue. I have never really mastered the art of plucking my eye brows. For those of you that did-good job! Again, a tip on how to do this and not have one eyebrow different than the other would have been nice. Well, while plucking my eye brows I found a grey hair! I never knew the eyebrows turned grey! I was started getting a few grey hairs at my scalp and I knew not to pluck because if you do one, seven come to the funeral. What to do about the grey eyebrow? I plucked it. Well, after that I found a grey hair down there! I was mortified! What do you do about that? That's when it hit me, I was aging. Well, you can't dye it. Remember the episode of *Sex and the City* when Samantha found a grey hair and dyed her lady parts? Well, it turned orange, I was not about to do that. Oh the shame and the realization I was getting older.

There is so much to talk about things that should be passed from one generation to another. I wonder if other generations just went through hell and thought, "I'm not going to tell anyone all the crap I am going through, let them figure it out." Did they just want us to go through the same hell? I don't have that answer, but believe me if I see my grandmothers in heaven, I am going to ask and say, "What the hell?!"

I Hate Aging

There are a few hard things in life that can make you feel really sad. Watching your parents and grandparents get older and decline in health is one of them. I don't remember my grandmothers taking care of great grandmas or my parents taking care of my grandparents. My great-grandparents died before my grandma could take care of them. I did help take care of one of my grandmothers at home before it was too much work and she was placed in a nursing facility. My step-grandparents had to be placed in nursing homes because of Alzheimer's disease. Now my parents and in-laws are aging, and boy is it tough to see them get older. You just don't think about it when you are younger. I didn't think that my dad would get old and fragile, but now after taking care of Gram, it is a sad reality.

My grandmother had dementia, as well as my step-grandparents, my step-mother, and my step uncle. It's so hard watching someone you love literally lose her mind. Sometimes I make jokes about it because my grandma did some pretty funny shit, and if she was in her right mind, she would've been so embarrassed. We used to play the guessing game. I would say, "What did you have for lunch?" (Her caregiver made her lunch.) She would say, "You know, what they have in San Francisco." I would say, "Oh, Rice-A-Roni®." That's from the old commercials: Rice-A-Roni®, the San Francisco treat. Or she would say, "CJ's favorite restaurant," which would be McDonald's®, my son's favorite place to eat. Super funny stuff. My step-grandma, Mimi, used to have these little dogs that barked all the time. Her very last words were, "Those damn dogs." She would always say that after they barked. She never spoke again, just opened her mouth as the staff fed her, dressed her, and cleaned her. Dementia is no laughing matter, but sometimes you have to laugh at the shit they do; it's the only way to not break down and cry. No one can prepare you for this. I can tell you that caring for a loved one is super hard, emotional, and physically exhausting. Watching a loved one—whether it's a person or fur family member—decline and die is super hard. No one can prepare you for this.

Is there a happy medium with aging? I guess you can be happy that you made it this far in life. I don't really want to get older, have the body changes and all the freaky shit in the middle that happens but I can't stop it. So, I must push past my stubborn self and try to embrace this season of my life.

Some Information Is Better Than Nothing

I can tell you a few things that my grandmothers and mothers did tell me. Some things can be helpful. My stepmom Rose did tell me a few times how to let things go, that "sticks and stones" type of mentality. I didn't always let it go though and got into a few fights, but hey, who didn't? As a young adult it hurts because we don't have that wisdom of letting things go, and some people are just plain mean and stupid. We haven't realized that'll never change and to just move on. She also said, "Beauty is as beauty does." I didn't understand it when I was younger, and I thought it was stupid. I understand now. Always treat others the way you want to be treated. That is so true. I remember always helping the special needs kids in school when others were mean to them. I felt no one should be mean to others, and to be honest I thought the other kids were being assholes just to treat people that way. To this day, I try really hard to remember that. Be polite and show respect to your elders. Treat others fairly. No matter how much you want to say what you really feel, don't. I think the younger generations need to remember this, because they currently do not. Always wash your makeup off your face before bed, and then apply moisturizer cream to your face and body. I have been doing that since I was about fourteen. Remember that skin is an organ, and you have to maintain it, or it will age before its time. It's okay to make mistakes. Learn from them and move on. Always do what feels right in your heart, whether it's related to a job, friends, or relationship. And never be mean to animals—I am a huge animal lover. (This has no relation to the topic, but I don't care.) When in doubt, ask questions, there is no shame in asking. Thank God every morning for waking to face another day and another challenge, and believing that all will be as it should. These are a few of the things I can remember. I think they are good, and hopefully you will too.

THE WRAP UP

In wrapping things up, I hope this had some good ideas to help you cope with life and the changes that you will go through or already have. Don't be afraid to ask your girlfriends questions. That's what they are there for. There is also the Internet now, which would have been super helpful when I was younger.

Well, there you have it. Life is outrageous. Some things would have been good to know to make it less cray cray. Maybe they wanted me to find out on my own maybe they thought it would be character building. Maybe I am a better person to find out life lessons on my own. Whatever the reason, I am finally feeling like I have some of the answers. That's what aging is all about, I suppose. The sucky thing is now that I am finally figuring it out my life is half-over. In my mind I still feel young, but my body has other plans. Try to enjoy the things that make you happy. Embrace life before you get too old to enjoy it. Travel, garden, love your family and friends…whatever makes you happy! But nothing that will cause harm to you or to others—ha-ha!

So, on my last note, remember that you are fabulous. It's okay to laugh at yourself. Embrace imperfections. Make mistakes and cherish the little things.

Cheers.

ABOUT THE AUTHOR

Mari F. Herman is a nurse manager with more than twenty years' experience in the nursing field. She has lived in the same town her whole life, is married with children and a dog, and looks for joy in everyday experiences.

www.ingramcontent.com/pod-product-compliance
Lightning Source LLC
Chambersburg PA
CBHW062025280526
45787CB00005B/2210